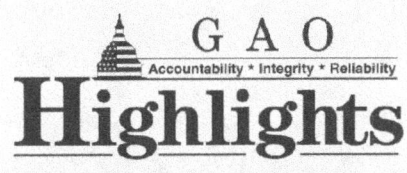

**GAO**
Accountability * Integrity * Reliability

# Highlights

Highlights of GAO-12-966, a report to congressional requesters

**September 2012**

## MEDICARE

### Higher Use of Advanced Imaging Services by Providers Who Self-Refer Costing Medicare Millions

## Why GAO Did This Study

Medicare Part B expenditures—which include payment for advanced imaging services—are expected to continue growing at an unsustainable rate. Questions have been raised about self-referral's role in this growth. Self-referral occurs when a provider refers patients to entities in which the provider or the provider's family members have a financial interest. GAO was asked to examine the prevalence of advanced imaging self-referral and its effect on Medicare spending. This report examines (1) trends in the number of and expenditures for self-referred and non-self-referred advanced imaging services, (2) how provision of these services differs among providers on the basis of whether they self-refer, and (3) implications of self-referral for Medicare spending. GAO analyzed Medicare Part B claims data from 2004 through 2010 and interviewed officials from the Centers for Medicare & Medicaid Services (CMS) and other stakeholders. Because Medicare claims lack an indicator identifying self-referred services, GAO developed a claims-based methodology to identify self-referred services and expenditures and to characterize providers as self-referring or not.

## What GAO Recommends

GAO recommends that CMS improve its ability to identify self-referral of advanced imaging services and address increases in these services. The Department of Health and Human Services, which oversees CMS, stated it would consider one recommendation, but did not concur with the others. GAO maintains CMS should monitor these self-referred services and ensure they are appropriate.

View GAO-12-966. For more information, contact James C. Cosgrove at (202) 512-7114 or cosgrovej@gao.gov.

## What GAO Found

From 2004 through 2010, the number of self-referred and non-self-referred advanced imaging services—magnetic resonance imaging (MRI) and computed tomography (CT) services—both increased, with the larger increase among self-referred services. For example, the number of self-referred MRI services increased over this period by more than 80 percent, compared with an increase of 12 percent for non-self-referred MRI services. Likewise, the growth rate of expenditures for self-referred MRI and CT services was also higher than for non-self-referred MRI and CT services.

GAO's analysis showed that providers' referrals of MRI and CT services substantially increased the year after they began to self-refer—that is, they purchased or leased imaging equipment, or joined a group practice that already self-referred. Providers that began self-referring in 2009—referred to as switchers—increased MRI and CT referrals on average by about 67 percent in 2010 compared to 2008. In the case of MRIs, the average number of referrals switchers made increased from 25.1 in 2008 to 42.0 in 2010. In contrast, the average number of referrals made by providers who remained self-referrers or non-self-referrers declined during this period. This comparison suggests that the increase in the average number of referrals for switchers was not due to a general increase in the use of imaging services among all providers. GAO's examination of all providers that referred an MRI or CT service in 2010 showed that self-referring providers referred about two times as many of these services as providers who did not self-refer. Differences persisted after accounting for practice size, specialty, geography, or patient characteristics. These two analyses suggest that financial incentives for self-referring providers were likely a major factor driving the increase in referrals.

**Change in Average Number of MRI Services Referred, 2008 and 2010**

|  | Average 2008 referred MRI services | Average 2010 referred MRI services | Percentage change |
|---|---|---|---|
| Switchers | 25.1 | 42.0 | 67.3 |
| Non-self-referrers | 20.6 | 19.2 | -6.8 |
| Self-referrers | 47.0 | 45.4 | -3.4 |

Source: GAO analysis of Medicare data.

Note: Pattern observed for MRI services was similar for CT services. GAO defines switchers as those providers that did not self-refer in 2007 or 2008, but did self-refer in 2009 and 2010.

GAO estimates that in 2010, providers who self-referred likely made 400,000 more referrals for advanced imaging services than they would have if they were not self-referring. These additional referrals cost Medicare about $109 million. To the extent that these additional referrals were unnecessary, they pose unacceptable risks for beneficiaries, particularly in the case of CT services, which involve the use of ionizing radiation that has been linked to an increased risk of developing cancer.

_____ **United States Government Accountability Office**

# Contents

Figures

## Abbreviations

| | |
|---|---|
| BETOS | Berenson-Eggers Type of Service |
| CMS | Centers for Medicare & Medicaid Services |
| CT | computed tomography |
| DRA | Deficit Reduction Act of 2005 |
| FFS | fee-for-service |
| HCPCS | Healthcare Common Procedure Coding System |
| HHS | Department of Health and Human Services |
| IDTF | independent diagnostic testing facility |
| MedPAC | Medicare Payment Advisory Commission |
| MRI | magnetic resonance imaging |
| NPI | national provider identifier |
| PC | professional component |
| PPACA | Patient Protection and Affordable Care Act |
| TC | technical component |
| TIN | taxpayer identification number |

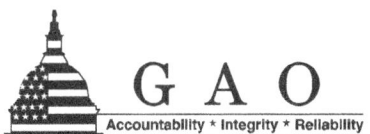

United States Government Accountability Office
Washington, DC 20548

September 28, 2012

Congressional Requesters

Expenditures for Medicare Part B services—which include physician and other outpatient services—are expected to continue exceeding the overall growth rate of the U.S. economy, heightening concerns about the long-range fiscal sustainability of Medicare.[1] While Medicare spending growth has slowed in recent years, expenditures for Medicare Part B grew by an average of 5.9 percent annually from 2007 through 2011 and are projected to grow by an average of 7.6 percent annually from 2012 through 2016.[2] In comparison, the national economy grew by an average annual rate of 2.5 percent from 2007 through 2011[3] and is projected to increase on average by 4.6 percent annually from 2012 through 2016.[4] Medicare Part B spending includes payments for advanced imaging services—magnetic resonance imaging (MRI) and computed tomography (CT) services—which providers use in the diagnosis and treatment of many diseases and disorders, such as different types of cancer, cardiovascular diseases, and musculoskeletal disorders.[5]

---

[1]Medicare is the federally financed health insurance program for persons aged 65 and over, certain individuals with disabilities, and individuals with end-stage renal disease. Medicare Part A covers hospital and other inpatient stays. Medicare Part B is optional insurance, and covers physician, outpatient hospital, home health care, and certain other services. Medicare Parts A and B are known as original Medicare or Medicare fee-for-service (FFS).

[2]See The Boards of Trustees, *2012 Annual Report of the Boards of Trustees of the Federal Hospital Insurance and Federal Supplementary Medical Insurance Trust Funds* (Washington, D.C.: April 2012). The projected Medicare Part B growth rate assumes that scheduled statutory cuts in physician payment rates will be overridden by Congress as they have been every year since 2003.

[3]See Bureau of Economic Analysis, "Gross Domestic Product (GDP) Percent change from preceding period," *National Economic Accounts* (Washington, D.C.: May 31, 2012), accessed June 27, 2012, http://www.bea.gov/national/xls/gdpchg.xls.

[4]See Congressional Budget Office, *The Budget and Economic Outlook: Fiscal Years 2012 through 2022* (Washington, D.C.: January 2012).

[5]Other advanced imaging services include nuclear medicine services. For the purposes of this report, "advanced imaging services" refers to only MRI and CT services.

Policymakers and researchers have raised questions about the growth in Part B spending, noting that some of this growth may be partially attributed to self-referral and that not all of the advanced imaging services provided may be appropriate or necessary.[6] Self-referral occurs when providers refer their patients to entities—such as themselves or a group practice—with which they or an immediate family member has a financial relationship, such as when a provider refers patients to his or her office for advanced imaging services after the provider purchases or leases advanced imaging equipment.[7] Proponents of self-referral point out that such arrangements allow providers to make rapid diagnoses, improve coordination of care, and provide convenient access for patients. However, critics of self-referral note that the incentive for financial gain in such arrangements may result in inappropriate, unnecessary, or potentially harmful services. For example, CT services expose beneficiaries to ionizing radiation, which is associated with an increased risk of cancer.

Growth in imaging services expenditures—including expenditures for advanced imaging services—have prompted action from Congress and resulted in recommendations from us and others. Specifically, Congress, as part of the Deficit Reduction Act of 2005 (DRA),[8] required that

---

[6]For example, see Laurence C. Baker, "Acquisition of MRI Equipment by Doctors Drives Up Imaging Use and Spending," *Health Affairs*, vol. 29, no. 12 (2010); Medicare Payment Advisory Commission, *Report to the Congress, Improving Incentives in the Medicare Program* (Washington, D.C.: June 2009); and Senator Grassley Press Release, *Grassley Works to Protect Medicare Dollars, Empower Patients with Information* (July 25, 2008), accessed May 31, 2012. http://www.finance.senate.gov/newsroom/ranking/release/?id=bb006ccf-dedc-40fd-9b14-6074cb2687f3.

[7]Compliance with the physician self-referral law, commonly known as the Stark law, is outside the scope of this report. The Stark law prohibits physicians from making referrals for certain designated health services paid for by Medicare, to entities with which the physicians or immediate family members have a financial relationship, unless the arrangement complies with a specified exception, such as in-office ancillary services. 42 U.S.C. § 1395nn(b)(2).The requirements of the in-office ancillary services exception are found at 42 C. F. R. § 411.355(b) (2011).The Patient Protection and Affordable Care Act (PPACA) amended the Stark law to establish an additional requirement with respect to the in-office ancillary services exception for certain types of advanced imaging services. That is, self-referring physicians must inform patients in writing at the time of referral for these services that the patient may obtain the service from a person other than the referring physician or someone in the physician's group practice and provide the patient with a list of suppliers who furnish the service in the area in which the patient resides. Pub. L. No. 111-148, § 6003, 124 Stat. 119, 697 (codified at 42 U.S.C. § 1395nn(b)(2)).

[8]Pub. L. No. 109-171, § 5102(b), 120 Stat. 4, 39-40 (2006).

Medicare payment for certain imaging services under the Medicare physician fee schedule—the payment system used to determine fees for physician-billed services in Medicare FFS—not exceed the amount Medicare pays under the hospital outpatient prospective payment system, used to pay for hospital outpatient services. In our 2008 report, we recommended that, to address the rapid growth in Medicare Part B imaging expenditures, the Centers for Medicare & Medicaid Services (CMS)—the agency within the Department of Health and Human Services that administers the Medicare program—examine the feasibility of expanding the use of front-end approaches for managing the utilization of advanced imaging services.[9] Front-end approaches to managing services are conducted prior to, rather than after, services are performed and payment is made. Examples of such approaches include requiring prior authorization (specific approval from a payer to perform a service) and privileging (limiting the authority to order certain services to only providers with specified qualifications). In contrast, back-end approaches are used after CMS issues payment, and could include targeted audits of providers that refer a high volume of services. Further, the Medicare Payment Advisory Commission (MedPAC) has recommended that certain providers with higher advanced imaging utilization participate in a prior authorization program and that CMS reduce payment rates for imaging services when the same provider orders and performs a service.[10] According to MedPAC, such a reduction would account for certain efficiencies that occur when the same provider orders and performs a service. Specifically, in these situations, the provider has likely already performed certain work involved in interpreting an imaging service, such as reviewing the patient's history, prior to making the referral. As of June 2012, CMS has not implemented MedPAC's or our recommendation.

You asked us to examine the prevalence of self-referral for advanced imaging services and Medicare spending for these services.[11] In this

---

[9]See GAO, *Medicare Part B Imaging Services: Rapid Spending Growth and Shift to Physician Offices Indicate Need for CMS to Consider Additional Management Practices*, GAO-08-452 (Washington, D.C.: June 13, 2008).

[10]See Medicare Payment Advisory Commission, *Report to the Congress: Medicare and the Healthcare Delivery System* (Washington, D.C.: June 2011).

[11]In addition to this report on advanced imaging, we also have ongoing work related to the self-referral of anatomic pathology services, intensity-modulated radiation therapy services, and physical therapy services.

report, we examine (1) trends in the number of and expenditures for self-referred and non-self-referred advanced imaging services from 2004 through 2010, (2) the extent to which the provision of advanced imaging services differs for providers who self-refer when compared with other providers, and (3) the implications of self-referral for Medicare spending on advanced imaging services.

To identify trends in the number of and expenditures for self-referred and non-self-referred advanced imaging services from 2004 through 2010, we analyzed claims from the Medicare Part B Carrier File for MRI and CT services.[12] Because there is no indicator or "flag" on the claim that identifies whether services are self-referred or non-self-referred and CMS has no other method for identifying whether a service was self-referred, we developed a claims-based methodology for identifying self-referred services.[13] Specifically, we classified services from the period we reviewed as self-referred if the provider that referred the beneficiary for a MRI or CT service and the provider that performed the MRI or CT service were identical or had a financial relationship with the same entity.[14] We removed MRI or CT services referred by radiologists or other providers that primarily practice in an independent diagnostic testing facility (IDTF) because they have limited ability to self-refer services.[15] We limited the universe for this portion of our analysis to those advanced imaging

---

[12]For the purposes of our report, we limited MRI or CT services (1) to those that were designated health services—services which, in the absence of an exception, a physician may not make a referral to furnish to an entity with which he has a financial relationship without implicating the Stark law—and (2) to those where the service includes the performance of the imaging service—which can be billed with or separately from the interpretation of a MRI or CT imaging service.

[13]An indicator or "flag" could be, for example, a modifier that a provider lists on a claim to indicate that a service is self-referred. Providers currently use modifiers to provide additional information about a service to CMS. For example, if a provider is only billing for the technical component of an imaging service, the provider would use a modifier to alert CMS that the claim does not cover the professional component of the service.

[14]Providers could have a financial relationship with the same entity if, for example, they are part of the same group practice.

[15]IDTFs are diagnostic testing facilities that are independent of a physician's office or hospital and that comply with a number of requirements including those related to the use of qualified supervising physicians, qualified nonphysician personnel, performance of only specifically ordered tests, and compliance with all applicable state laws. See 42 C.F.R. § 410.33 (2011). Radiologists and providers in IDTFs predominantly perform advanced imaging services and have limited ability to refer beneficiaries for advanced imaging services. These providers are unlikely to self-refer MRI or CT services.

services performed in a provider's office or in an IDTF, which represents approximately one-fifth of all advanced imaging services provided to Medicare FFS beneficiaries.[16] Providers in our analysis include primarily physicians, but could include other providers, such as nurse practitioners and physician assistants. We focused on services performed in these settings because our previous work showed rapid growth among such services and because the financial incentive for providers to self-refer is most direct when the service is performed in a physician office. We used the claims to identify trends in the number and proportion of self-referred and non-self-referred MRI and CT services performed from 2004 through 2010, the expenditures for these services from 2004 through 2010, and the proportion of self-referred and non-self-referred MRI and CT services by provider specialty for 2004 and 2010. To determine expenditures, we used the allowed charges variable from the Medicare Part B Carrier File, which includes the amounts paid by Medicare and the beneficiary.

To determine the extent to which the provision of advanced imaging services differed for providers who self-refer when compared with other providers, we performed two separate analyses. First, we compared the provision—that is, the number of referrals made—of MRI and CT services by self-referring providers and non-self-referring providers in 2010, after accounting for factors such as practice size (i.e., the number of Medicare beneficiaries), provider specialty, geography (i.e., urban or rural), and patient characteristics.[17] For this analysis, our universe of providers included all those providers that referred at least one MRI or CT service, except for providers that had a specialty of radiology, emergency medicine, or provided services in an IDTF.[18] Second, we determined the extent to which the number of MRI and CT referrals made by providers changed after they began to self-refer. Specifically, we identified a group

---

[16]Providers can also provide advanced imaging services in settings other than physician offices or IDTFs, such as hospitals.

[17]We defined urban areas as metropolitan statistical areas, a geographic entity defined by the Office of Management and Budget as a core urban area of 50,000 or more population; all other settings are considered rural.

[18]Providers with a radiology or IDTF specialty were removed because they have limited ability to refer beneficiaries for advanced imaging services, and thus are not likely to self-refer MRI or CT services. We excluded emergency medicine providers from our analysis because they did not practice in provider offices. After we made our exclusions, there were 419,884 providers that referred at least one MRI service and 477,547 providers that referred at least one CT service in 2010.

of providers that began to self-refer advanced imaging services in 2009. We then calculated the change in the number of MRI or CT referrals made from 2008 (i.e., the year before they began self-referring) to 2010 (i.e., the year after they began self-referring). We compared the change in the number of referrals made by these providers to the change in the number of referrals made over the same time period by providers who did not change whether or not they self-referred advanced imaging services. We classified providers as self-referring if they self-referred at least one MRI or CT service and non-self-referring if they referred—but did not self-refer—at least one MRI or CT service.[19] For both analyses we counted all services that a provider referred, regardless of whether it was performed in a provider office, IDTF, or other setting, such as a hospital.

To determine the implications of self-referral for Medicare spending on advanced imaging services, we estimated what Medicare expenditures under the physician fee schedule for self-referred advanced imaging services would have been in 2010 if the rate of referrals made by self-referring providers equaled the rate of referrals made by providers who did not self-refer. We compared this to the actual expenditures under the physician fee schedule, using the allowed charges variable, for self-referred advanced imaging services of the same specialty and provider size and calculated the difference. To ensure comparisons were meaningful, we limited this analysis to providers in those specialties that had at least 1,000 self-referring providers.[20]

We took several steps to ensure that the data used to produce this report were sufficiently reliable. Specifically, we assessed the reliability of the CMS data we used by interviewing officials responsible for overseeing these data sources, reviewing relevant documentation, and examining the data for obvious errors. We determined that the data were sufficiently reliable for the purposes of our study. (See app. I for more details on our scope and methodology.)

---

[19]In 2010, 35,950 providers self-referred an MRI service and 39,913 providers self-referred a CT service. In comparison, there were 383,934 non-self-referring MRI providers and 437,634 non-self-referring CT providers.

[20]We defined physician specialty using the specialty codes included in the Medicare claims. These specialty codes include physician specialties, such as cardiology and hematology/oncology, and nonphysician provider types, such as nurse practitioners and physician assistants.

We conducted this performance audit from May 2010 through September 2012 in accordance with generally accepted government auditing standards. Those standards require that we plan and perform the audit to obtain sufficient, appropriate evidence to provide a reasonable basis for our findings and conclusions based on our audit objectives. We believe that the evidence obtained provides a reasonable basis for our findings and conclusions based on our audit objectives.

## Background

MRI and CT services are two types of medical imaging that aid in the diagnosis and treatment of myriad diseases and disorders. Medicare reimburses providers for performing the services and, subsequently, interpreting the results. Payment for the performance of the service can be made through different payment systems, depending on where the service is performed. In 2010, 6.8 million MRI and CT services were performed in a physician office or IDTF, representing about 23 percent of all MRI and CT services received by Medicare FFS beneficiaries. CMS has implemented several policies to limit self-referral, and MedPAC and other researchers have proposed further reforms.

## MRI and CT Services

Medical imaging is a noninvasive process used to obtain pictures of the internal anatomy or function of the anatomy using one of many different types of imaging equipment and media for creating the image. MRI and CT services are two of the six medical imaging modalities.[21] MRI services use magnets, radio waves, and computers to create images of internal body tissues. CT services use ionizing radiation and computers to produce cross-sectional images of internal organs and body structures. For certain advanced imaging services, contrast agents, such as barium or iodine solutions, are administered to patients orally or intravenously. By using contrast, sometimes referred to as "dye," as part of the imaging examination, providers can view soft tissue and organ function more clearly. MRI and CT services help diagnose and treat many diseases and disorders such as different types of cancer, cardiovascular diseases, and musculoskeletal disorders. They can also reduce the need for more-invasive medical procedures and improve patient outcomes.

---

[21]The other four imaging modalities are nuclear medicine, ultrasound, X-ray and other standard imaging, and procedures that use imaging.

| Medicare Billing and Payment Policies for Advanced Imaging Services | Medicare payments for advanced imaging services are separated into two components—the technical component (TC) and the professional component (PC). The TC is intended to cover the cost of performing a test, including the costs for equipment, supplies, and nonphysician staff. The PC is intended to cover the provider's time in interpreting the image and writing a report on the findings. The PC and TC can be billed together, on what is called a global claim. The components can also be billed separately. For instance, a global claim could be billed if the same provider performs and interprets the examination, whereas the TC and PC could be billed separately if the performing and interpreting providers are different. Typically, the Medicare payment for the TC is substantially higher than the payment for the PC. For instance, for a CT of the pelvis with dye billed under the 2010 Medicare physician fee schedule, the TC accounted for 79 percent of the total payment, and the PC accounted for 21 percent. |
|---|---|
| | Medicare reimburses providers through different payment systems depending on where the advanced imaging service is performed. When an advanced imaging service is performed in a provider's office or an IDTF, both the PC and TC are reimbursed under the Medicare physician fee schedule. Alternatively, when the service is performed in an institutional setting, such as a hospital outpatient or inpatient department, the provider is reimbursed under the Medicare physician fee schedule for the PC, while the TC is reimbursed under a different Medicare payment system, according to the setting in which the service was provided. For instance, the TC of an advanced imaging service performed in a hospital outpatient department is reimbursed under the Medicare hospital outpatient payment system, while a service performed in a hospital inpatient setting is reimbursed through a facility payment paid under Medicare Part A. |

| 2010 Advanced Imaging Utilization by Setting and Medicare Physician Fee Schedule Expenditures | In 2010, Medicare FFS beneficiaries received 30.0 million advanced imaging services, approximately 6.8 million (23 percent) of which were performed in an IDTF or physician's office. Of the 6.8 million advanced imaging services performed in an IDTF or physician's office, 2.9 million were MRI services and 3.9 million were CT services. The remaining 23.2 million advanced imaging services were performed in other settings, such as hospital inpatient or outpatient departments, and their associated TCs were billed through different payment systems (see fig. 1). The total expenditures for all advanced imaging services billed under the Medicare physician fee schedule, including TCs and PCs, reached $4.2 billion in 2010. |
|---|---|

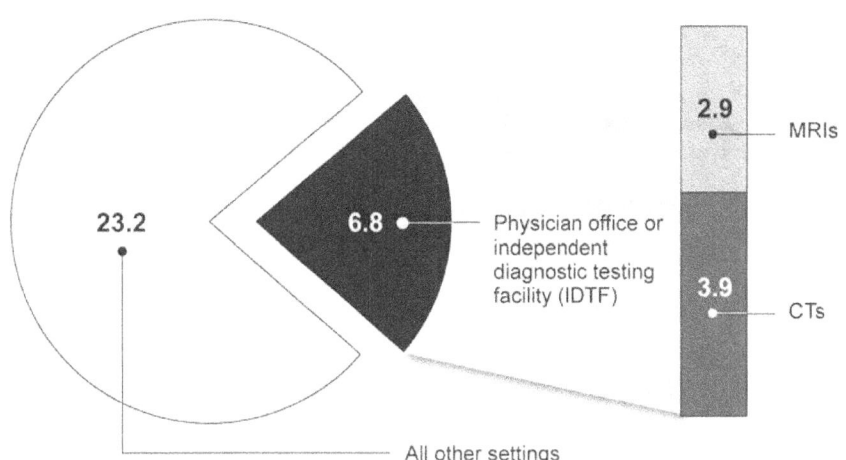

Figure 1: Distribution of Advanced Imaging Services by Modality and Setting, 2010

Number of services (in millions)

23.2

6.8 — Physician office or independent diagnostic testing facility (IDTF)

2.9 — MRIs

3.9 — CTs

All other settings

Source: GAO analysis of Medicare data

## Select Implemented or Proposed Policies Designed to Address Utilization or Expenditures Associated with Self-Referral of Advanced Imaging Services

Numerous policies have been implemented or proposed by CMS, MedPAC, or other researchers that are designed to limit self-referral or reduce inappropriate utilization of advanced imaging services. These policies can affect self-referral or advanced imaging utilization through various means such as prohibiting different types of physician self-referral, informing beneficiaries of physician self-referral, mandating accreditation of staff performing MRI and CT services, improving payment accuracy, reducing payments for self-referred services, and ensuring services are clinically appropriate. One type of physician self-referral arrangement that CMS has prohibited is "per-click" self-referral arrangements where, for instance, a physician leases an imaging machine to a hospital, refers patients for imaging services, and then is paid on a per-service basis by the hospital. CMS has also solicited comments on prohibiting self-referral of diagnostic tests provided as an ancillary service in a physician's office that are not usually provided during an office visit, because a key rationale for permitting self-referral of such services is that receiving a diagnostic service during the same office visit when a physician orders a test is convenient for beneficiaries. MedPAC, in its June 2010 report to Congress, noted that MRI and CT services were performed on the same day as an office visit less than a quarter of the time, with only 8.4 percent of MRI services of the brain being performed on the same day as an office visit.[22] Appendix II lists a select number of such policies in addition to these two policies that have been implemented or put forth by CMS, MedPAC, and other researchers.

## Self-Referred MRI and CT Services and Expenditures Grew Overall, While Non-Self-Referred Services and Expenditures Grew Slower or Decreased

From 2004 through 2010, the number of self-referred MRI and CT services performed in a provider's office and non-self-referred MRI and CT services performed in a provider's office or IDTF increased, with the larger increase for self-referred services. Similarly, expenditures for self-referred advanced imaging services also increased over this period, and this increase was larger than the changes in expenditures for advanced imaging services that were not self-referred. Over the period we reviewed, the share of advanced imaging services that were self-referred also increased overall and across all provider specialties we examined.

## Number of Self-Referred and Non-Self-Referred MRI and CT Services Increased Overall from 2004 to 2010, with the Larger Increase among Self-Referred Services

While the number of self-referred MRI services performed in a provider's office and non-self-referred MRI services performed in a provider's office or IDTF both increased from 2004 through 2010, a significantly larger increase occurred among the self-referred services.[23] Specifically, the number of self-referred MRI services increased from about 380,000 services in 2004 to about 700,000 services in 2010—an increase of more than 80 percent (see fig 2). In contrast, the number of non-self-referred MRI services grew about 12 percent over the same time period, from about 1.97 million services in 2004 to about 2.21 million services in 2010. Despite an overall increase during this time, both self-referred and non-self-referred services declined at some point during the years of our study. However, the number of self-referred services grew faster in the

---

[22]Medicare Payment Advisory Commission, *Report to Congress: Aligning Incentives in Medicare* (Washington, D.C.: June 2010).

[23]As noted in the Scope and Methodology section, the universe of services for this finding refers to advanced imaging services performed in a provider's office or in an IDTF. We focused on these settings because our previous work showed rapid growth among such services and because the financial incentive for providers to self-refer is most direct when the service is performed in a physician office.

earlier years and declined less in the later years than the number of non-self-referred services.

**Figure 2: Number of Self-Referred and Non-Self-Referred MRI Services, 2004-2010**

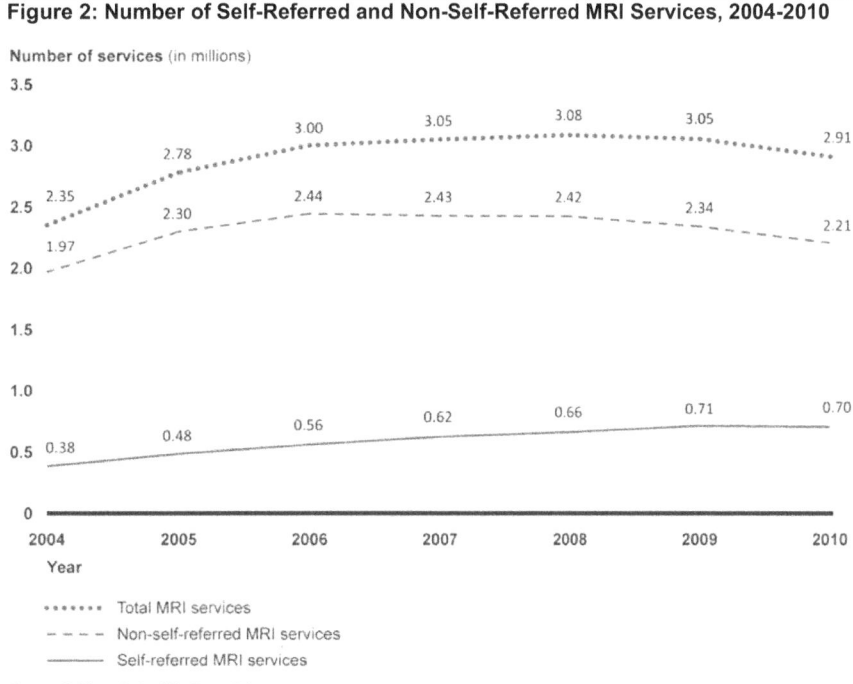

Number of services (in millions)

Source: GAO analysis of Medicare data

Note: Results include services performed in a physician office or IDTF. Services performed in other settings, such as hospital outpatient departments, are not included.

Similar to MRI services, the number of self-referred and non-self-referred CT services both increased from 2004 through 2010, with a considerably larger increase occurring in self-referred services. Specifically, the number of self-referred CT services more than doubled from 2004 through 2010, growing from about 700,000 services to about 1.45 million services (see fig. 3). In contrast, the number of non-self-referred CT services increased about 30 percent during these years, from about 1.90 million services to about 2.48 million services. Although the number of both self-referred and non-self-referred CT services increased over the period of our study, the number of non-self-referred CT services decreased from 2009 through 2010.

**Figure 3: Number of Self-Referred and Non-Self-Referred CT Services, 2004-2010**

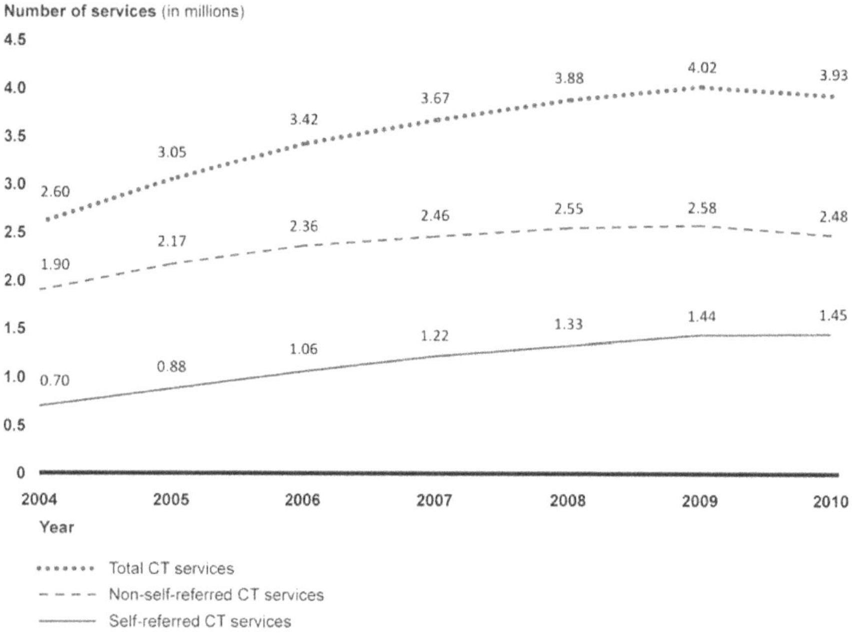

Number of services (in millions)

```
••••••  Total CT services
– – – –  Non-self-referred CT services
———  Self-referred CT services
```

Source: GAO analysis of Medicare data

Note: Results include services performed in a physician office or IDTF. Services performed in other settings, such as hospital outpatient departments, are not included.

The number of self-referred advanced imaging services increased from 2004 through 2010, even after accounting for change in the number of Medicare FFS beneficiaries. Specifically, the number of self-referred MRI services per 1,000 Medicare FFS beneficiaries grew from 10.8 in 2004 to 20.0 in 2010—an increase of about 85 percent. Similarly, the number of self-referred CT services per 1,000 Medicare FFS beneficiaries more than doubled, growing from about 19.6 in 2004 to 41.2 in 2010.

## Self-Referred MRI and CT Expenditures Grew More Than Non-Self-Referred Expenditures Overall with Non-Self-Referred MRI Expenditures Declining

Expenditures for self-referred MRI services grew overall from 2004 through 2010, while expenditures for non-self-referred MRI services declined. Specifically, self-referred MRI expenditures grew about 55 percent during the time of our review, from approximately $239 million in 2004 to about $370 million in 2010 (see fig. 4). In contrast, expenditures for non-self-referred MRI services decreased about 8.5 percent during the same period. Expenditures for both self-referred and non-self-referred MRI services increased rapidly from 2004 through 2006, then decreased sharply in 2007. These declines in 2007 corresponded with the first year of implementation of a DRA provision that reduced fees for certain advanced imaging services.[24] Since the declines in 2007, expenditures for non-self-referred MRI services have declined further while self-referred expenditures have increased.

---

[24]Under a provision in the DRA, Medicare fees for certain imaging services covered by the Medicare physician fee schedule cannot exceed what Medicare pays under the hospital outpatient prospective payment system, effectively mandating reduction in fees for certain services. Pub. L. No. 109-171, § 5102(b), 120 Stat. 4, 39-40 (2006). See GAO, *Medicare: Trends in Fees, Utilization, and Expenditures for Imaging Services before and after Implementation of the Deficit Reduction Act of 2005*, GAO-08-1102R (Washington, D.C.: September 26, 2008).

**Figure 4: Self-Referred and Non-Self-Referred MRI Expenditures, 2004-2010**

Expenditures (in millions of dollars)

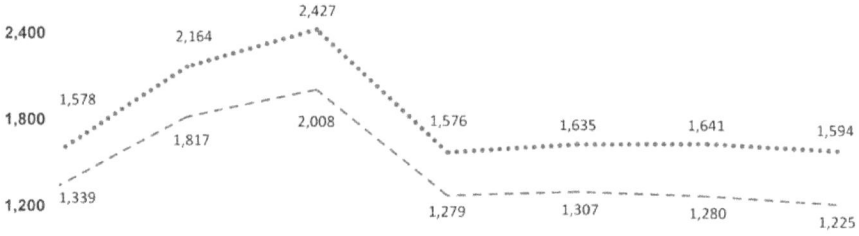

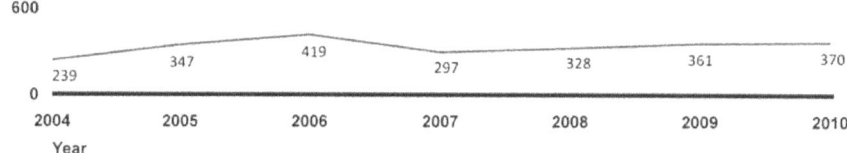

....... Total expenditures

– – – – Non-self-referred MRI expenditures

——— Self-referred MRI expenditures

Source: GAO analysis of Medicare data.

Note: Expenditures include those services we could determine were performed in a physician office or IDTF setting. This included global claims where the performance and interpretation of the advanced imaging service were billed together—and claims where the performance of the advanced imaging service was billed separately from the interpretation of the image. We excluded expenditures for claims where the interpretation of the exam was billed separately because this service may have been performed in another setting, such as a hospital outpatient department.

Relative to 2004, expenditures for both self-referred and non-self-referred CT services have grown through 2010, but the increase was larger for self-referred CT services (see fig. 5). Specifically, expenditures for self-referred CT services increased from $204 million in 2004 to about $340 million in 2010, an increase of about 67 percent. In contrast, expenditures for non-self-referred CT services increased from about $609 million in 2004 to about $642 million in 2010, an increase of about 5 percent.

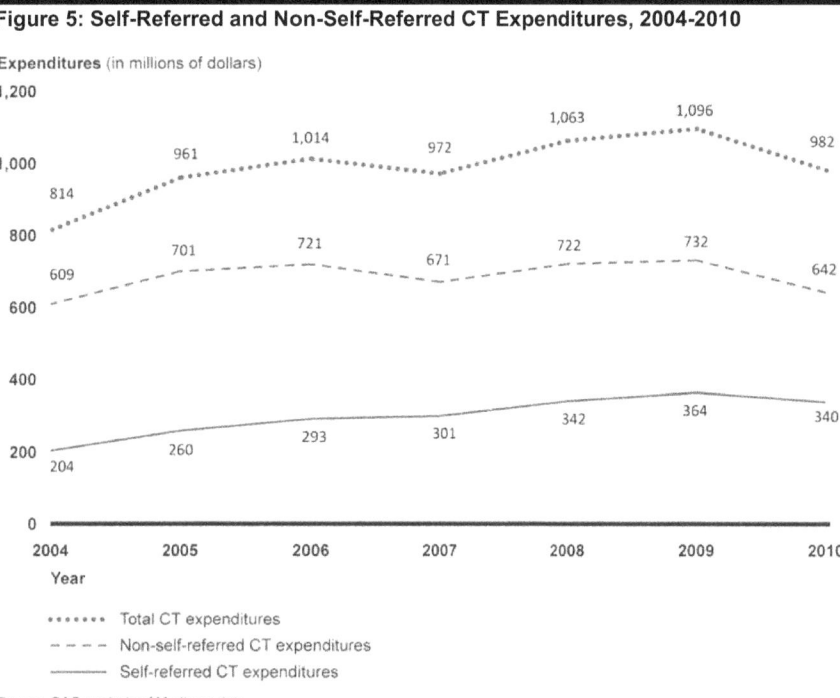

Figure 5: Self-Referred and Non-Self-Referred CT Expenditures, 2004-2010

Source: GAO analysis of Medicare data

Note: Expenditures include those services we could determine were performed in a physician office or IDTF setting. This included global claims where the performance and interpretation of the advanced imaging service were billed together—and claims where the performance of the advanced imaging service was billed separately from the interpretation of the image. We excluded expenditures for claims where the interpretation of the exam was billed separately because this service may have been performed in another setting, such as a hospital outpatient department.

## Share of Self-Referred MRI and CT Services Increased Overall and across All Major Referring Provider Specialties

Because the self-referred advanced imaging services grew at a greater rate than non-self-referred services from 2004 through 2010, the proportion of MRI and CT services that were self-referred increased during that time period. Specifically, the proportion of MRI services that were self-referred increased from 16.3 percent in 2004 to 24.2 percent in 2010. Similarly, the proportion of CT services that were self-referred grew from 26.8 percent in 2004 to 37.0 percent in 2010. Consistent with the overall trend, the proportion of MRI and CT services that were self-referred increased from 2004 through 2010 for all provider specialties that we studied.[25] For further information on self-referral rates across provider specialties, see appendix III.

## Self-Referring Providers Referred Substantially More Advanced Imaging Services on Average Than Did Other Providers

We found that, in 2010, providers that self-referred beneficiaries for MRI and CT services referred substantially more of those services than did providers who did not self-refer these services, even after we accounted for differences in practice size, specialty, geography, and patient characteristics. We also found that the year after providers purchased MRI or CT equipment, leased MRI or CT equipment, or joined a group practice that self-referred, they increased the number of services they referred when compared with providers that did not begin to self-refer advanced imaging services.

### Self-Referring Providers Referred Substantially More MRI and CT Services Than Other Providers, Regardless of Practice or Patient Characteristics

In 2010, self-referring providers referred substantially more advanced imaging services than providers who did not self-refer such services that year.[26] Specifically, providers that self-referred at least one beneficiary for an MRI service in 2010 averaged 36.4 MRI referrals, compared with an average of 14.4 MRI referrals for non-self-referrers. Similarly, providers that self-referred at least one beneficiary for a CT service in 2010 averaged 73.2 CT referrals, or 2.3 times as many as the 32.3 CT referrals averaged by non-self-referring providers. About 10 percent of all MRI and CT services referred by self-referring providers in 2010 were ordered, performed, and interpreted by the same provider. Certain efficiencies may be gained when the same provider orders, performs, and interprets an advanced imaging service, such as reviewing a patient's clinical history only once. CMS has taken steps to ensure that fees for services paid under the physician fee schedule take into account efficiencies that

[25]We included specialties that referred at least 1.5 percent of self-referred MRI or CT services in 2004 and 2010. Sixteen provider specialties met these criteria for MRI services, CT services, or both types of services. These specialties were Cardiology, Family Practice, Gastroenterology, General Surgery, Hematology/Oncology, Internal Medicine, Medical Oncology, Neurology, Neurosurgery, Physical Medicine, Pulmonary Disease, Orthopedic Surgery, Otolaryngology, Radiation Oncology, Rheumatology, and Urology.

[26]As discussed earlier, the scope of services included in this analysis is broader than our analysis of self-referred services. Specifically, this analysis includes settings other than a physician office or IDTF, such as a hospital. We did this to fully capture the advanced imaging referral patterns of self-referring and non-self-referring providers to ensure that the comparison between the groups was comparable.

resulted from how the services are provided, and we recently recommended that CMS expand these efforts.[27]

Differences in advanced imaging referrals between self-referring and non-self-referring providers persisted after accounting for differences in practice size, specialty, geography, or patient characteristics.

## Practice Size

Self-referring providers referred more MRI and CT services than did non-self-referring providers, regardless of differences in practice size. In general, self-referring providers tend to work in practices with a larger number of Medicare beneficiaries. However, in 2010, self-referring providers referred more MRI and CT services than non-self-referring providers regardless of practice size, and the difference in number of services referred generally increased as provider size increased (see table 1). For example, self-referring providers that had 50 or fewer patients referred 1.8 times as many MRI services as did non-self-referring providers. In comparison, self-referring providers with 500 or more patients referred 2.4 times as many MRI services as non-self-referring providers did.

---

[27]CMS has a long-standing policy called a multiple procedure payment reduction that is meant to avoid duplicate payments for expenses that are incurred only once when two or more surgical services are furnished together by the same physician during the same operating session. CMS expanded the multiple procedure payment reduction to include certain imaging services in 2006. Medicare Program: Revisions to Payment Policies Under the Physician Fee Schedule for Calendar Year 2006, 70 Fed. Reg. 70116 (Nov. 21, 2005). In our 2009 report, we recommended that CMS expand its efforts to ensure that fees for services paid under the physician fee schedule reflect efficiencies that occur when services are performed by the same physician to the same beneficiary on the same day. See GAO, *Medicare Physician Payments: Fees Could Better Reflect Efficiencies Achieved When Services Are Provided Together*, GAO-09-647 (Washington, D.C.: July 31, 2009). In 2012, CMS expanded its multiple procedure payment reduction policy by applying a reduction to the PC of imaging services that are provided during the same session, to the same patient, on the same day; the agency had previously applied the multiple procedure payment reduction to only the TC of imaging services that met the same criteria.

**Table 1: Average Number of MRI and CT Services Referred by Non-Self-Referring and Self-Referring Providers, 2010**

| Number of unique Medicare FFS beneficiaries[a] | MRI services | | | CT services | | |
|---|---|---|---|---|---|---|
| | Non-self-referring | Self-referring | Relative rate of self-referring providers[b] | Non-self-referring | Self-referring | Relative rate of self-referring providers[b] |
| 1 to 50 | 3.2 | 5.7 | 1.8 | 5.2 | 7.1 | 1.4 |
| 51 to 100 | 7.2 | 12.3 | 1.7 | 13.7 | 19.0 | 1.4 |
| 101 to 250 | 13.0 | 24.0 | 1.8 | 26.7 | 40.8 | 1.5 |
| 251 to 500 | 20.4 | 42.8 | 2.1 | 48.7 | 78.8 | 1.6 |
| >500 | 29.7 | 71.1 | 2.4 | 89.9 | 151.0 | 1.7 |

Source: GAO analysis of Medicare data.

Notes: Providers were considered to be self-referring if they self-referred beneficiaries for at least one service. Providers with a specialty of radiology or independent diagnostic testing facility (IDTF) were removed from this analysis because they should not be able to self-refer services. Additionally, because emergency medicine providers generally did not practice in provider offices, they were removed from our analysis. Of the 419,884 providers that referred at least one beneficiary for an MRI service in 2010, 35,950 were self-referring and 383,934 were non-self-referring. Of the 477,547 providers that referred at least one beneficiary for a CT service in 2010, 39,913 were self-referring and 437,634 were non-self-referring.

[a]The number of unique Medicare FFS beneficiaries refers to the number of unique beneficiaries that received at least one service from a provider.

[b]The relative rate of self-referring providers refers to the factor by which the average number of services referred by self-referring providers is greater than the average number of services referred by non-self-referring providers. For example, if the relative rate of self-referring providers is equal to 3, it would mean that, on average, self-referrers refer 3 times as many advanced imaging services as do non-self-referrers.

## Specialty

Self-referring providers generally referred more MRI and CT services than did non-self-referring providers, regardless of differences in specialties. Self-referring providers were more likely than non-self-referring providers to belong to specialties that had a greater-than-average number of referrals per physician for advanced imaging services in 2010. However, for the 7 specialties that had at least 1,000 providers that self-referred beneficiaries for MRI services, self-referring providers generally averaged more referrals for MRI services than did non-self-referring providers, regardless of practice size.[28] Similarly, self-referring providers in 9 of the

---

[28]We grouped providers of each specialty with at least 1,000 self-referring providers into five provider-size categories: (1) fewer than 50 unique Medicare FFS patients; (2) 51-100 unique Medicare FFS patients; (3) 101-250 unique Medicare FFS patients; (4) 251-500 unique Medicare FFS patients; and (5) more than 500 unique Medicare FFS patients. The seven specialties that had at least 1,000 self-referring providers were Family Practice, Hematology/Oncology, Internal Medicine, Neurology, Nurse Practitioners, Orthopedic Surgeons, and Physician Assistants.

13 specialties that had at least 1,000 self-referring CT providers generally referred more beneficiaries for CT services than non-self-referring providers, regardless of practice size.[29]

## Geography

Self-referring providers referred more MRI and CT services than non-self-referring providers, regardless of differences in geography. Providers that self-referred MRI services averaged 36.3 MRI referrals and 37.3 MRI referrals in urban and rural locations, respectively. In comparison, non-self-referring providers averaged 14.3 MRI referrals in urban locations and 15.2 MRI referrals in rural locations. Providers that self-referred beneficiaries for CT services averaged 72.7 referrals in urban locations and 77.2 referrals in rural locations, while non-self-referring providers averaged 31.1 CT referrals in urban locations and 40.7 referrals in rural locations. We found that differences in the number of MRI and CT referrals made by self-referring and non-self-referring providers persisted when accounting for provider size along with geography (see table 2).

[29]The nine specialties where self-referring providers referred more beneficiaries for CT services than non-self-referring providers across the majority of provider size categories were: Cardiology, Gastroenterology, General Surgery, Hematology/Oncology, Nurse Practitioners, Orthopedic Surgery, Otolaryngology, Urology, and Pulmonary Disease specialists. The four specialties where non-self-referring providers referred more beneficiaries for CT services, on average, than self-referring providers across the majority of provider size categories were Family Practice, Internal Medicine, Neurology, and Physician Assistants.

**Table 2: Average Number of MRI and CT Services Referred by Non-Self-Referring and Self-Referring Providers in Urban and Rural Locations, 2010**

| Geographic designation | Number of unique Medicare FFS beneficiaries[a] | MRI services | | | CT services | | |
|---|---|---|---|---|---|---|---|
| | | Non-self-referring | Self-referring | Relative rate of self-referring providers[b] | Non-self-referring | Self-referring | Relative rate of self-referring providers[b] |
| Urban | 1 to 50 | 3.3 | 5.8 | 1.8 | 5.4 | 7.3 | 1.4 |
| | 51 to 100 | 7.5 | 12.4 | 1.7 | 14.2 | 19.4 | 1.4 |
| | 101 to 250 | 13.5 | 24.4 | 1.8 | 27.2 | 41.9 | 1.5 |
| | 251 to 500 | 20.8 | 43.9 | 2.1 | 48.2 | 80.8 | 1.7 |
| | >500 | 29.5 | 72.1 | 2.4 | 86.5 | 151.5 | 1.8 |
| Rural | 1 to 50 | 2.8 | 4.7 | 1.7 | 4.3 | 5.2 | 1.2 |
| | 51 to 100 | 5.7 | 10.2 | 1.8 | 10.4 | 12.7 | 1.2 |
| | 101 to 250 | 10.5 | 20.1 | 1.9 | 23.8 | 30.3 | 1.3 |
| | 251 to 500 | 19.0 | 34.6 | 1.8 | 51.3 | 64.7 | 1.3 |
| | >500 | 30.5 | 65.4 | 2.1 | 102.8 | 147.8 | 1.4 |

Source: GAO analysis of Medicare data.

Notes: Providers were considered to be self-referring if they self-referred beneficiaries for at least one service. Providers with a specialty of radiology or independent diagnostic testing facility (IDTF) were removed from this analysis because they should not be able to self-refer services. Additionally, because emergency medicine providers generally did not practice in provider offices, they were removed from our analysis. Of the 419,884 providers that referred at least one beneficiary for an MRI service in 2010, 35,950 were self-referring and 383,934 were non-self-referring. Of the 477,547 providers that referred at least one beneficiary for a CT service in 2010, 39,913 were self-referring and 437,634 were non-self-referring.

[a]The number of unique Medicare FFS beneficiaries refers to the number of unique beneficiaries that received at least one service from a provider.

[b]The relative rate of self-referring providers refers to the factor by which the average number of services referred by self-referring providers is greater than the average number of services referred by non-self-referring providers. For example, if the relative rate of self-referring providers is equal to 3, it would mean that, on average, self-referrers refer 3 times as many advanced imaging services as do non-self-referrers.

## Patient Characteristics

Self-referring providers referred more MRI and CT services than non-self-referring providers, in spite of similarities in patient characteristics. Specifically, the patient populations of self-referring and non-self-referring MRI and CT providers were similar in terms of most patient characteristics, with self-referring providers having slightly healthier patients than non-self-referring providers, as indicated by their lower average risk score (see table 3). If self-referring providers had patients that were older or sicker, it could have explained why self-referring providers referred their patients for more services than non-self-referring providers.

GAO-12-966 Medicare Self-Referral of Advanced Imaging Services

**Table 3: Patient Characteristics of Non-Self-Referring and Self-Referring MRI and CT Providers, 2010**

| Patient characteristics, average | MRI services | | CT services | |
|---|---|---|---|---|
| | Non-self-referring | Self-referring | Non-self-referring | Self-referring |
| Average age (years) | 70 | 71 | 70 | 71 |
| Percent female | 59 | 60 | 59 | 57 |
| Average risk score[a] | 1.53 | 1.40 | 1.57 | 1.44 |

Source: GAO analysis of Medicare data.

[a]A beneficiary's risk score is a proxy for health status and is equivalent to the ratio of expected health care expenditures for that beneficiary under Medicare FFS relative to the average health care expenditures for all Medicare FFS beneficiaries. For example, a beneficiary with a risk score of 1.05 would have expected expenditures that were 5 percent higher than an average Medicare FFS beneficiary. The risk scores presented are normalized using the FFS normalization factor of 1.041 that CMS used to normalize risk scores in 2010. Normalization keeps the average Medicare FFS risk score constant at 1.0 over time.

## Providers' Referrals for MRI and CT Services Substantially Increased the Year after They Began to Self-Refer

Our analysis indicated that providers' referrals for MRI and CT services substantially increased the year after they began to self-refer. In our analysis, we compared the number of MRI and CT referrals for switchers—those providers that did not self-refer in 2007 or 2008 but did self-refer in 2009 and 2010—to providers that did not change their self-referral status during the same time period. Providers could self-refer by purchasing imaging equipment, leasing equipment, or joining a group practice that already self-referred. Overall, the switcher group of providers who began self-referring in 2009 increased the average number of MRI and CT referrals they made by about 67 percent in 2010 compared to the average in 2008. In the case of MRIs, the average number of referrals switchers made for MRI services increased from 25.1 in 2008 to 42.0 in 2010. In contrast, the average number of MRI and CT referrals declined for providers that did not self-refer and providers who self-referred from 2008 through 2010. This comparison suggests that the increase in the average number of referrals for switchers from 2008 to 2010 was not due to a general increase in the use of imaging services among all providers. (See table 4.)

**Table 4: Change in Average Number of MRI and CT Services Referred, 2008 and 2010**

| Provider referral type | MRI Services | | | | CT Services | | | |
|---|---|---|---|---|---|---|---|---|
| | Number of providers | Average 2008 referred MRI services | Average 2010 referred MRI services | Percentage change, 2008 to 2010 | Number of providers | Average 2008 referred CT services | Average 2010 referred CT services | Percentage change, 2008 to 2010 |
| Switchers | 2,803 | 25.1 | 42.0 | 67.3 | 3,329 | 56.3 | 93.9 | 66.7 |
| Non-self-referrers | 199,102 | 20.6 | 19.2 | -6.8 | 241,097 | 59.1 | 58.1 | -1.7 |
| Self-referrers | 17,753 | 47.0 | 45.4 | -3.4 | 19,756 | 89.6 | 87.3 | -2.6 |

Source: GAO analysis of Medicare data.

Note: We define switchers as those providers that did not self-refer in 2007 or 2008, but did self-refer in 2009 and 2010.

The increase in MRI and CT referrals for providers that began self-referring in 2009 cannot be explained exclusively by factors such as providers joining practices with higher patient volumes, different patient populations, or different practice cultures. Specifically, providers that remained in the same practice from 2007 through 2010, but began self-referring in 2009, also had a bigger increase in the number of MRI and CT referrals than did providers that did not change their self-referral status.[30] Providers that remained in the same practice from 2008 through 2010, but began self-referring in 2009 had a 21.0 percent increase in MRI referrals and a 14.4 percent increase in CT referrals.

## Higher Use of Advanced Imaging Services by Self-Referring Providers Results in Substantial Costs to Medicare

On the basis of our estimates, Medicare spent about $109 million more in 2010 than the program would have if self-referring providers referred advanced imaging services at the same rate as non-self-referring providers of the same specialty and provider size (see fig. 6). This additional spending can be attributed to the fact that self-referring providers referred over 400,000 more MRI and CT services in 2010 than if they had referred at the same rate as non-self-referring providers of the same size and specialty. Specifically, we estimate there were 143,303 additional referrals for MRI services and 283,725 additional referrals for CT services.

---

[30]We considered a provider to have remained in the same practice if the entity to which they most commonly referred MRI or CT services remained the same from 2007 through 2010.

**Figure 6: Potential Savings under Alternative Scenario for Self-Referring Providers, 2010**

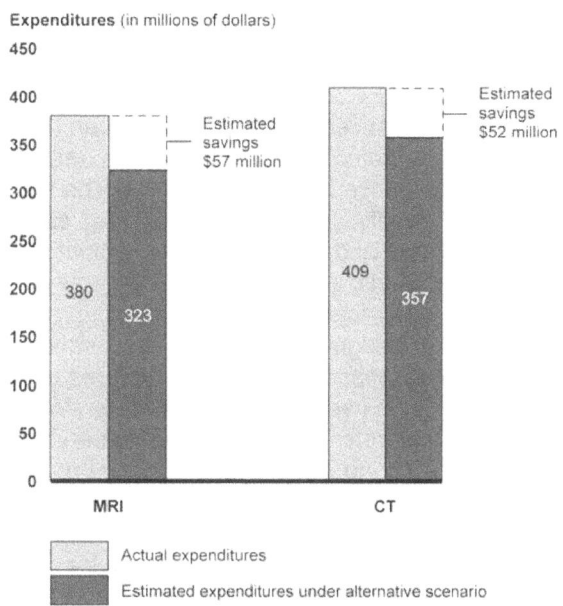

Expenditures (in millions of dollars)

Actual expenditures

Estimated expenditures under alternative scenario

Source: GAO analysis of Medicare data

Note: We included imaging expenditures for those specialties that had at least 1,000 self-referring providers. Overall, specialties that met these criteria referred approximately 66 percent of self-referred MRI services and approximately 81 percent of self-referred CT services. Under the alternative scenario, we calculated expenditures for services as if self-referring providers referred MRI and CT services at the same rate as non-self-referring providers of the same specialty and practice size in 2010.

The additional Medicare imaging expenditures attributed to self-referring providers is likely higher than $109 million in 2010.[31] This is because a significant portion of self-referring providers are not included in this estimate. Specifically, we limited our analysis to those specialties that had at least 1,000 self-referring providers. Approximately 34 percent of the

---

[31]We limited our analysis to expenditures directly related to imaging services. There may be additional costs associated with the increased use of advanced imaging services by self-referring providers, if these imaging services reveal abnormalities that have no clinical relevance or result in unnecessary surgeries. In contrast, increased use of advanced imaging may partially offset some of these direct imaging costs if increased use led to the early detection of disease and resulted in less-invasive and less-costly treatments.

providers who self-referred beneficiaries for MRI services and 19 percent of the providers who self-referred beneficiaries for CT services belonged to a specialty other than those that met the 1,000 self-referring providers criteria.

## Conclusions

Advanced imaging services can help in the early detection and aid in the treatment of certain diseases, resulting in less-invasive treatments and improved patient outcomes. The ability of providers to self-refer beneficiaries for these services can, for example, improve coordination of care and help ensure convenient access to these services among beneficiaries. However, our review indicates that some factor or factors other than the health status of patients, provider practice size or specialty, or geographic location (i.e., rural or urban) helped drive the higher advanced imaging referral rates among self-referring providers compared to non-self-referring providers. We found that providers who began to self-refer advanced imaging services—after purchasing or leasing imaging equipment or joining practices that self-referred—substantially increased their referrals for MRI and CT services relative to other providers. This suggests that financial incentives for self-referring providers may be a major factor driving the increase in referrals. These financial incentives likely help explain why, in 2010, providers who self-referred made 400,000 more referrals for advanced imaging services than they would have if they were not self-referring. These additional referrals cost CMS more than $100 million in 2010 alone. To the extent that these additional referrals are unnecessary, they pose an unacceptable risk for beneficiaries, particularly in the case of CT services, which involve the use of ionizing radiation.

Given the challenges to the long-range fiscal sustainability of Medicare, it is imperative that CMS develop policies to address the effect of self-referral on the utilization of and expenditures for advanced imaging services. CMS first needs to improve its ability to identify services that are self-referred. Claims do not include an indicator or "flag" that identifies whether services are self-referred or non-self-referred, and CMS does not currently have a method for easily identifying such services. A systematic method for identifying self-referred advanced imaging services would give CMS the ongoing ability to determine the extent to which these services are self-referred and help the agency identify those services that may be inappropriate, unnecessary, or potentially harmful to beneficiaries. Including a self-referral flag on Medicare Part B claims submitted by providers who bill for advanced imaging services is likely the easiest and most cost-effective approach. Second, we found that about 10 percent of advanced imaging services referred by self-referring physicians in 2010 were also performed and interpreted by the same physician. Certain efficiencies may be gained when the same provider orders, performs, and interprets an advanced imaging service, such as reviewing a patient's clinical history only once. MedPAC recommended in 2011 that CMS should reduce its payments for advanced imaging services in which the same provider refers and performs the service, to account for efficiencies that are realized in these circumstances. This is consistent with previous efforts by CMS to reduce fees for services paid under the physician fee schedule when efficiencies are realized and with our previous recommendation that CMS expand these efforts. Third, if CMS were able to easily identify self-referred services, the agency may be better positioned to implement an approach that ensures the appropriateness of advanced imaging services that Medicare beneficiaries receive—beyond examining the feasibility of such methods, as we recommended in our 2008 report. Approaches for managing advanced imaging utilization could be "front-end" or used before CMS issues payment, such as prior authorization. CMS could also explore back-end approaches used after CMS issues payment, such as targeted audits of self-referring providers that refer a high volume of services.

## Recommendations for Executive Action

In order to improve CMS's ability to identify self-referred advanced imaging services and help CMS address the increases in these services, we recommend that the Administrator of CMS take the following three actions:

1. Insert a self-referral flag on its Medicare Part B claims form and require providers to indicate whether the advanced imaging services for which a provider bills Medicare are self-referred or not.

2. Determine and implement a payment reduction for self-referred advanced imaging services to recognize efficiencies when the same provider refers and performs a service.

3. Determine and implement an approach to ensure the appropriateness of advanced imaging services referred by self-referring providers.

## Agency Comments and Our Evaluation

HHS reviewed a draft of this report and provided written comments, which are reprinted in appendix IV. In its comments, HHS stated that it would consider one of our recommendations but did not concur with our other two recommendations. HHS did not comment on our findings that self-referring providers referred substantially more advanced imaging services than non-self-referring providers or our conclusion that financial incentives for self-referring providers may be a major factor driving the increase in referrals for advanced imaging services.

HHS noted that it would consider our recommendation that CMS determine and implement an approach to ensure the appropriateness of advanced imaging services referred by self-referring providers. According to HHS, CMS would consider this recommendation when refining its medical review strategy for advanced imaging services. HHS also indicated that CMS does not have statutory authority to implement some of the approaches discussed in the report. We are pleased that CMS plans to consider this recommendation and note that we did not identify a specific approach, having identified several examples in our report of both front-end and back-end approaches to managing utilization of advanced imaging services. As we reported, CMS could explore back-end approaches used after CMS issues payment, such as targeted audits of self-referring providers. CMS could also explore other approaches the agency determines are within its statutory authority. Further, if deemed necessary, CMS could seek legislative authority to implement promising approaches to managing advanced imaging utilization.

HHS did not concur with our recommendation that CMS insert a self-referral flag on its Medicare Part B claims and require providers to indicate whether the advanced imaging services for which a provider bills Medicare are self-referred or not. According to HHS, CMS believes that a new checkbox on the claim form identifying self-referral would be complex to administer and providers may not characterize referrals accurately. CMS believes that other payment reforms, such as paying networks of providers, hospitals, or other entities that share responsibility for providing care to patients, would better address overutilization. We continue to believe that including an indicator or flag on the claims would likely be the easiest and most cost-effective approach to improve CMS's ability to identify self-referred advanced imaging services. We do not suggest, nor did we intend, that CMS use the self-referral flag or indicator we recommended to determine compliance with the physician self-referral law. Without a self-referral flag or indicator, CMS will not be able to monitor trends in utilization and expenditures associated with physician self-referral without considerable time and effort. Further, a self-referral flag does not have to be a "checkbox" on the claim and could be a modifier, similar to other modifiers that CMS uses to characterize claims. In addition, HHS did not provide reasons to support CMS's contention that such a flag would be complex to administer.

HHS also did not concur with our recommendation that CMS determine and implement a payment reduction for self-referred advanced imaging services to recognize efficiencies when the same provider refers and performs a service. According to HHS, CMS's multiple procedure payment reduction already captures efficiencies inherent in providing multiple advanced imaging services by the same physician or group practice during the same session. CMS also noted that a further payment reduction may reduce, but not eliminate, the underlying financial incentive to self-refer advanced imaging services and may cause providers to refer more services, in an effort to maintain their income. CMS also noted that providers in a group practice could easily avoid this reduction by having one physician order the service while another furnishes the service. According to HHS, CMS also questions its statutory authority to impose the payment reduction for the subset of physicians who self-refer, citing a prohibition on paying a differential by physician specialty for the same service. Our report shows that self-referring providers generally referred more MRI and CT services, regardless of differences in specialties, and CMS did not indicate how this recommendation would implicate the prohibition on paying a differential by specialty. Additionally, while HHS cites the multiple procedure payment reduction as a means to address certain efficiencies in the delivery of advanced imaging services, these are not the efficiencies targeted by our recommendation. Instead, as noted in our report, our recommended payment reduction would capture those efficiencies gained when the same provider orders and performs an advanced imaging service. Such efficiencies could be captured in a single—rather than multiple—advanced imaging service. This recommendation is also consistent with a 2011 MedPAC recommendation. As noted in our report, this payment reduction would affect about 10 percent of advanced imaging services referred by self-referring providers. As for CMS's concern about overutilization of advanced imaging services resulting from a payment reduction, CMS could help address this issue by implementing our recommendation to use a flag indicating self-referral to monitor utilization of these services.

On the basis of HHS's written response to our report, we are concerned that neither HHS nor CMS appears to recognize the need to monitor the self-referral of advanced imaging services on an ongoing basis and determine those services that may be inappropriate, unnecessary, or potentially harmful to beneficiaries. HHS did not comment on our key finding that self-referring physicians referred about two times as many advanced imaging services, on average, as providers who did not self refer. Nor did HHS comment on our estimate that these additional referrals for advanced imaging services cost CMS more than $100 million in 2010 alone. Given these findings, we continue to believe that CMS should take steps to monitor the utilization of advanced imaging services and ensure that the services for which Medicare pays are appropriate.

HHS also provided technical comments that we incorporated as appropriate.

As agreed with your offices, unless you publicly announce the contents of this report earlier, we plan no further distribution until 30 days from the report date. At that time, we will send copies to the Secretary of HHS, interested congressional committees, and others. In addition, the report will be available at no charge on the GAO website at http://www.gao.gov.

If you or your staff has any questions about this report, please contact me at (202) 512-7114 or cosgrovej@gao.gov. Contact points for our Offices of Congressional Relations and Public Affairs may be found on the last page of this report. GAO staff who made major contributions to this report are listed in appendix V.

James C. Cosgrove
Director, Health Care

*List of Requesters*

The Honorable Max Baucus
Chairman
Committee on Finance
United States Senate

The Honorable Chuck Grassley
Ranking Member
Committee on the Judiciary
United States Senate

The Honorable Henry A. Waxman
Ranking Member
Committee on Energy and Commerce
House of Representatives

The Honorable Sander Levin
Ranking Member
Committee on Ways and Means
House of Representatives

The Honorable Pete Stark
Ranking Member
Subcommittee on Health
Committee on Ways and Means
House of Representatives

# Appendix I: Scope and Methods

This section describes the scope and methodology used to analyze our three objectives: (1) trends in the number of and expenditures for self-referred and non-self-referred advanced imaging services from 2004 through 2010, (2) the extent to which the provision of advanced imaging services differs for providers who self-refer when compared with other providers, and (3) the implications of self-referral for Medicare spending on advanced imaging services.

For all three objectives, we used the Medicare Part B Carrier File, which contains final action Medicare Part B claims for noninstitutional providers, such as physicians. Claims can be for one or more services or for individual service components.[1] Each service or service component is identified on a claim by its Healthcare Common Procedure Coding System (HCPCS) code, which the Centers for Medicare & Medicaid Services (CMS) assigns to products, supplies, and services for billing purposes. HCPCS codes are also categorized by CMS using the Berenson-Eggers Type of Service (BETOS) categorization system, which assigns HCPCS to broad service categories.[2]

We limited our universe of services and service components for our study to those for magnetic resonance imaging (MRI) and computed tomography (CT) services. We classified MRI and CT services and service components as those with HCPCS codes included in a BETOS category where the first two digits were equal to "I2", defined as advanced imaging services. We further limited our universe to only those MRI and CT services that were considered designated health services—services for which, in the absence of an exception, a physician may not make a referral to furnish to an entity with which he has a financial relationship

---

[1]Services can have technical components (TC) and professional components (PC). The TC of a service is intended to cover the performance of a test, including the cost of equipment, supplies, and nonphysician staff. In addition, services have a PC, which for advanced imaging services is intended to cover the physician's time in interpreting an image and writing a report on the findings. The TC and PC of a service can be billed together on the same claim—called a global claim—or separately.

[2]The BETOS categorization system was developed by CMS primarily for analyzing the growth in Medicare expenditures by broad categories. Each billing code is assigned to only one BETOS category.

without implicating the Stark law.[3] Annually, CMS publishes a list of designated health services as part of the physician fee schedule. We also restricted our universe to those HCPCS codes that involved the performance of an advanced imaging service, which can be billed with or separately from the interpretation of a MRI or CT imaging service. We identified 125 HCPCS codes that met these criteria.

Because there is no indicator or "flag" on the claim that identifies whether services were self-referred or non-self-referred, we developed a claims-based methodology for identifying self-referred services. Specifically, we classified services as self-referred if the provider that referred the beneficiary for a MRI or CT service and the provider that performed the MRI or CT service was identical or had a financial relationship with the same entity. We used taxpayer identification number (TIN), an identification number used by the Internal Revenue Service, to determine providers' financial relationships. The TIN could be that of the provider, the provider's employer, or another entity to which the provider reassigns payment.[4] In order to identify the associated TINs for the referring and performing providers, we created a crosswalk of the performing provider's unique physician identification number or national provider identifier (NPI)

---

[3]Compliance with the physician self-referral law, commonly known as the Stark law, is outside the scope of this report. The Stark law prohibits physicians from making referrals for certain designated health services paid for by Medicare, to entities with which the physicians or immediate family members have a financial relationship, unless the arrangement complies with a specified exception, such as in-office ancillary services. 42 U.S.C. § 1395nn(b)(2).

[4]Some providers may be associated with TINs with which they do not have a direct or indirect financial relationship and thus would not have the same incentives as other self-referring providers. We anticipate that relatively few providers in our self-referring group meet this description but to the extent that they do, it may have limited the differences we found in utilization and expenditure rates between self-referring and non-self-referring providers.

to the TIN that appeared on the claim and used that to assign TINs to the referring and performing providers.[5]

We considered global services and separately-billed TCs to be self-referred if one or more of the TINs of the referring and performing provider matched. However, we did not consider separately-billed PCs to be self-referred, even if they met the same criterion. Compared to the payment for the TC of an advanced imaging service, the payment for the PC is relatively small, and thus there is little incentive for providers to only self-refer the PC of a service. As part of developing this claims-based methodology to identify self-referred services, we interviewed officials from CMS, provider groups, and other researchers.

To describe the trends in the number of and expenditures for self-referred and non-self-referred advanced imaging services from 2004 through 2010, we used the Medicare Part B Carrier File to calculate utilization and expenditures for self-referred and non-self-referred MRI and CT services, both in aggregate and per beneficiary. We limited this portion of our analysis to global claims or claims for a separately-billed TC, which indicates that the performance of the imaging service was billed under the physician fee schedule. As a result, the universe for this portion of our analysis are those advanced imaging services performed in a provider's office or in an independent diagnostic testing facility (IDTF), which both bill for the performance of an advanced imaging service under the physician fee schedule. We focused on these settings because our previous work showed rapid growth among such services and because the financial incentive for providers to self-refer is most direct when the service is performed in a physician office. Approximately one-fifth of all

---

[5]The final rule implementing the Health Insurance Portability and Accountability Act established the standard for a unique health identifier for health care providers for use in the health care system and announced the adoption of the NPI as that standard. HIPAA Administrative Simplification: Standard Unique Health Identifier for Health Care Providers, 69 Fed. Reg. 2424 (Jan. 23, 2004) (adding a new subpart D to 45 C.F.R. part 162). Performing physicians were required to include their NPI on any claim submitted to Medicare as of May 23, 2008. Prior to implementation of the NPI, Medicare required providers to submit another type of unique provider identifier called the unique physician identification number.

Our methodology for identifying self-referred services was similar to the methodology used by MedPAC for its study of the effect of physician self-referral on use of imaging services within an episode. See Medicare Payment Advisory Commission: *Report to the Congress: Improving Incentives in the Medicare Program* (Washington, DC, June 2009).

advanced imaging services provided to Medicare FFS beneficiaries were performed in a physician office or IDTF. To calculate the number of Medicare beneficiaries from 2004 through 2010 needed for per beneficiary calculations, we used the Denominator File, a database that contains enrollment information for all Medicare beneficiaries enrolled in a given year. Because radiologists and IDTFs are limited in their ability to generate referrals for advanced imaging services, we removed services referred by an IDTF or radiologist.

To determine the extent to which the provision of advanced imaging services differs for providers who self-refer when compared with other providers, we first classified providers on the basis of the type of referrals they made. Specifically, we classified providers as self-referring if they self-referred at least one beneficiary for an advanced imaging service.[6] We classified providers as non-self-referring if they referred a beneficiary for an advanced imaging service, but did not self-refer any of the services. Because radiologists and providers in IDTFs predominantly perform advanced imaging services and have limited ability to refer beneficiaries for advanced imaging services, we removed those providers from our analysis. Additionally, because emergency medicine providers generally did not practice in provider offices, they were removed from our analysis. We assigned to each provider the MRI and CT service and service-components that he or she referred, including those for the performance of an imaging service and those for the interpretation of the imaging service result. If the TC and PC were billed separately for the same beneficiary, we counted these two components as one referred service. As a result, we counted all services that a provider referred, regardless of whether it was performed in a provider office, IDTF, or other setting. We then performed two separate analyses.

First, we compared the provision—that is, the number of referrals made—of MRI and CT services by self-referring providers and non-self-referring providers in 2010, after accounting for factors such as practice size (i.e., the number of Medicare beneficiaries), provider specialty, geography (i.e., urban or rural), and patient characteristics. We used the number of unique Medicare fee-for-service (FFS) beneficiaries for which providers provided services in 2010 as a proxy for practice size, which we identified

---

[6]Providers in our analysis that could self-refer include primarily physicians, but also could include other providers, such as nurse practitioners and physician assistants.

using 100 percent of providers' claims from the Medicare Part B Carrier File. We defined urban settings as metropolitan statistical areas, a geographic entity defined by the Office of Management and Budget as a core urban area of 50,000 or more population. We used rural-urban commuting area codes—a Census tract-based classification scheme that utilizes the standard Bureau of Census Urbanized Area and Urban Cluster definitions in combination with work-commuting information to characterize all of the nation's Census tracts regarding their rural and urban status—to identify providers as practicing in metropolitan statistical areas.[7] We considered all other settings to be rural. We identified providers' specialties on the basis of the specialties listed on the claims. These specialty codes include physician specialties, such as cardiology and hematology/oncology, and nonphysician provider types, such as nurse practitioners and physician assistants. We also examined the extent to which the characteristics of the patient populations served by self-referring and non-self-referring providers differed. We used CMS's risk score file to identify average risk score, which serves as a proxy for beneficiary health status. Information on additional patient characteristics, such as age and sex, came from the Medicare Part B Carrier File claims. To calculate the percentage of advanced imaging services referred by self-referring providers that were referred, performed, and interpreted by the same provider, we summed global advanced imaging claims where the referring and performing provider were the same and claims where the TC and PC were referred and performed separately for the same beneficiary by the same provider. We then divided the total by the number MRI and CT services referred by self-referring providers.

Second, we determined the extent to which the number of MRI and CT referrals made by providers changed after they began to self-refer. Specifically, we identified a group of providers that began to self-refer advanced imaging services in 2009.[8] We refer to this group of providers as "switchers" because it represents providers that did not self-refer in 2007 or 2008, but did self-refer in 2009 and 2010. We then calculated the change in the number of MRI or CT referrals made from 2008 (i.e., the

---

[7]We considered a location with a rural-urban commuting area code of 1.0, 1.1, 2.0, 2.1, or 3.0 to be a metropolitan statistical area.

[8]We used 4 years of experience (2007 through 2010) to categorize providers even though we compared referrals in 2008 to 2010 because we wanted to ensure that providers that began self-referring in 2009 did not self-refer for at least the 2 prior years.

year before the switchers began self-referring) to 2010 (i.e., the year after they began self-referring). We compared the change in the number of referrals made by these providers to the change in the number of referrals made over the same time period by providers who did not change whether or not they self-referred advanced imaging services. Specifically, we compared the change in the number of referrals made by switchers to those made by (1) self-referring providers—providers that self-referred in years 2007 through 2010, and (2) non-self-referring providers—providers that did not self-refer in years 2007 through 2010. For each provider, we also identified the most common TIN to which they referred MRI or CT services. If the TIN was the same for all 4 years, we assumed that they remained part of the same practice for all 4 years. We calculated the number of referrals in 2008 and 2010 separately for providers that met this criterion.

To determine the implications of self-referral for Medicare spending on advanced imaging services, we summed the number of and expenditures for all MRI and CT services performed in 2010 by providers of those specialties with at least 1,000 self-referring providers. We then created an alternative scenario in which self-referring providers referred the same number of services as non-self-referring providers of the same provider size and specialty and calculated how this affected expenditures. To do this, we calculated the number of advanced imaging services non-self-referring providers referred per unique Medicare FFS beneficiary for each specialty and practice size. We then multiplied the referral rate times the number of patients seen by self-referring providers of the same practice size and specialty, representing the number of services self-referring providers would have referred if they referred at the non-self-referring rate. To calculate the cost of additional services to Medicare, we multiplied the difference between the self-referred services and the number of services they would have referred if they referred at the same rate as non-self-referring providers by the average expenditures for a MRI or CT service.

We took several steps to ensure that the data used to produce this report were sufficiently reliable. Specifically, we assessed the reliability of the CMS data we used by interviewing officials responsible for overseeing these data sources, reviewing relevant documentation, and examining the data for obvious errors. We determined that the data were sufficiently reliable for the purposes of our study.

We conducted this performance audit from May 2010 through September 2012 in accordance with generally accepted government auditing standards. Those standards require that we plan and perform the audit to obtain sufficient, appropriate evidence to provide a reasonable basis for our findings and conclusions based on our audit objectives. We believe that the evidence obtained provides a reasonable basis for our findings and conclusions based on our audit objectives.

# Appendix II: Select Implemented or Proposed Policies Designed to Address Self-Referral or the Utilization of Advanced Imaging Services

| Policy approach | Description and examples of policies |
|---|---|
| Informing Beneficiaries of Physician Self-Referral | Effective January 1, 2011, the Patient Protection and Affordable Care Act of 2010 (PPACA) requires physicians who self-refer MRI, CT, or positron emission tomography services under certain circumstances to inform their patients that they may obtain these services from another provider and provide their patients with a list of alternative providers in their area.[a]<br><br>The effect of this requirement on physician self-referral is unclear. The American College of Radiology reports that multiple states had similar requirements in place before the implementation of PPACA.[b] |
| Mandating Accreditation of Staff Performing MRI and CT Services | In 2008, the Centers for Medicare and Medicaid (CMS) proposed, but did not adopt, a requirement that provider office-based imaging practices enroll as independent diagnostic testing facilities (IDTF).[c] However, the Medicare Improvements for Patients and Providers Act of 2008 requires physicians and other providers to be accredited by a CMS-approved national accreditation organization by January 1, 2012, in order to continue to furnish the technical component of services such as MRI and CT services.[d] While the intent of this requirement was to improve quality of care, this policy could reduce the number of providers who self-refer if they fail to gain accreditation. However, this policy's actual effect on self-referral is unclear. |
| Improving Payment Accuracy | The Medicare Payment Advisory Commission (MedPAC) has noted that improving the payment accuracy of services could reduce the incentive to self-refer those services by making them less financially beneficial.[e] Consistent with our previous recommendations, payment rates for MRI and CT services have been reduced several times over the last few years to reflect efficiencies that occur when the same provider performs multiple services on the same patient on the same day.[f,g] |
| Reducing Payments for Physician Self-Referred Services | In its June 2010 report, MedPAC noted that reducing payments for physician self-referred services could limit Medicare expenditures when self-referral occurs and reduce the incentive to self-refer by making it less financially beneficial.[h] One option put forth in the report is reducing payments for certain self-referred services by an amount equal to the percent expenditures increase due to self-referral. Another option discussed is reducing the payment for self-referred services when they include activities already performed by self-referring physicians, such as reviewing the medical history of a beneficiary. |
| Ensuring Services are Clinically Appropriate | In addition to a similar recommendation from MedPAC, we have recommended CMS consider expanding its front-end management capabilities, such as prior authorization— an approach whereby providers must seek some sort of approval before ordering an advanced imaging service.[i,j] Such policies could limit the increased utilization associated with self-referral by ensuring that self-referred services are clinically appropriate.<br><br>One researcher suggested expanding postpayment reviews by making imaging a subject for medical review by recovery audit contractors.[k,l] |

**Appendix II: Select Implemented or Proposed
Policies Designed to Address Self-Referral or
the Utilization of Advanced Imaging Services**

| Policy approach | Description and examples of policies |
|---|---|
| Prohibiting Different Types of Physician Self-Referral | CMS has prohibited different types of physician self-referral that the agency deemed particularly susceptible to abuse. Effective October 1, 2009, CMS prohibits "per-click" self-referral arrangements where, for instance, a physician leases an imaging machine to a hospital, refers patients to that hospital in order to receive imaging services, and then is paid on a per service basis by the hospital.[m]<br><br>In 2008, CMS considered but did not prohibit "block time" self-referral arrangements where, for instance, a physician leases a block of time on a facility's MRI or CT machine, refers his or her patients to receive services on the facility's machine, and then bills for the services.[n]<br><br>CMS has also solicited comments on a prohibition against physician self-referral for diagnostic tests provided in physician offices when those tests are not needed at the time of a patient's office visit in order to assist the physician in determining an appropriate diagnosis or plan of treatment.[o] MedPAC has found that MRI and CT services are performed on the same day as an office visit less than a quarter of the time, with only 8.4 percent of MRIs of the brain being performed on the same day as an office visit.[p]<br><br>Another policy, discussed in MedPAC's June 2010 report, that would limit physician self-referral is restricting certain types of self-referral to only those practices that are clinically integrated.<br><br>Maryland prohibits providers from making self-referrals for certain MRI and CT services.[q] |

Source: GAO analysis of select self-referral regulations and proposals.

[a]Pub. L. No. 11-148, § 6003, 124 Stat. 199, 697.

[b]American College of Radiology, *State-by-State Comparison of Physician Self-Referral Laws*, accessed July 26, 2010.

[c]Medicare Program; Revisions to Payment Policies Under the Physician Fee Schedule and Other Revisions to Part B for CY 2009, 73 Fed. Reg. 38502, 28533 (July 7, 2008).

[d]Pub. L. No. 110-275, §135(a), 122 Stat. 2494, 2532.

[e]See Medicare Payment Advisory Commission, *Report to Congress: Aligning Incentives in Medicare* (Washington, D.C.: June 2010).

[f]See GAO, *Medicare Physician Payments: Fees Could Better Reflect Efficiencies Achieved When Services Are Provided Together*, GAO-09-647 (Washington, D.C.: July 31, 2009).

[g]For instance, in 2006, CMS began reducing the payment for the technical component of the lower-priced imaging service by 25 percent when multiple services are performed on contiguous body parts during the same session. See Medicare Program: Revisions to Payment Policies Under the Physician Fee Schedule for Calendar Year 2006, 70 Fed. Reg. 70116 (Nov. 21, 2005). PPACA increased the payment reduction from 25 percent to 50 percent beginning July 1, 2010. Pub. L. No. 111-148, §3135(b), 124 Stat. 119, 437. CMS also expanded this policy beginning January 1, 2012 by reducing payments for the lower-priced professional component of advanced imaging services by 25 percent when two or more services are furnished by the same physician to the same patient, in the same session, on the same day.

[h]See Medicare Payment Advisory Commission, *Report to Congress: Aligning Incentives in Medicare* (Washington, D.C.: June 2010).

[i]See Medicare Payment Advisory Commission, *Report to the Congress: Medicare and the Healthcare Delivery System* (Washington, D.C.: June 2011).

[j]See GAO, *Medicare Part B Imaging Services: Rapid Spending Growth and Shift to Physician Offices Indicate Need for CMS to Consider Additional Management Practices*, GAO-08-452 (Washington, D.C.: June 13, 2008).

[k]Donald H. Romano, "Self-Referral of Imaging and Increased Utilization: Some Practical Perspectives on Tackling the Dilemma," *Journal of the American College of Radiology* (2009): 773-779.

**Appendix II: Select Implemented or Proposed
Policies Designed to Address Self-Referral or
the Utilization of Advanced Imaging Services**

lThe stated goal of the recovery audit program is to identify improper payments for services provided to Medicare beneficiaries. Improper payments may be overpayments or underpayments. Overpayments can occur when health care providers submit claims that do not meet Medicare's coding or medical necessity policies.

mMedicare Program; Changes to Disclosure of Physician Ownership in Hospitals and Physician Self-Referral Rules, 73 Fed. Reg. 48434, 48713 (Aug. 19, 2008).

nMedicare Program; Changes to Disclosure of Physician Ownership in Hospitals and Physician Self-Referral Rules, 73 Fed. Reg. 48434, 48719 (Aug. 18, 2008).

oMedicare Program; Proposed Revisions to Payment Policies Under the Physician Fee Schedule, and Other Part B Payment Policies for CY 2008, 72 Fed. Reg. 38122, 38181 (July 12, 2007).

pSee Medicare Payment Advisory Commission, *Report to Congress: Aligning Incentives in Medicare* (Washington, D.C.: June 2010).

qMd. Code Ann., Health Occ. § 1-301(k)(2).

# Appendix III: Self-Referral of MRI and CT Services, by Provider Specialty, in 2004 and 2010

The proportion of MRI services and CT services that were self-referred increased from 2004 through 2010 for all provider specialties we examined for our study. We examined all provider specialties that performed a minimum proportion of either self-referred MRI or CT services in 2004 and 2010.[1] While this increase across provider specialties is consistent with the overall trend of increased self-referral, the increases varied among provider specialties. For MRI services, increases in the self-referral rate for provider specialties ranged from about 4 percentage points (Internal Medicine) to about 19 percentage points for Hematology/Oncology. Similarly, for CT services, increases in the self-referral rates for provider specialties ranged from about 2 percentage points (Internal Medicine) to over 38 percentage points (Radiation Oncology). (see table 5).

---

[1]Specifically, for MRI and CT services, we examined provider specialties that referred at least 1.5 percent of the MRI or CT services that were self-referred in both 2004 and 2010. Specialties we examined referred about 86 percent of self-referred MRI services in 2004 and about 81 percent of self-referred MRI services in 2010. These specialties referred about 82 percent of self-referred CT services in 2004 and about 88 percent of self-referred CT services in 2010.

Appendix III: Self-Referral of MRI and CT
Services, by Provider Specialty, in 2004 and
2010

Table 5: Self-referral Rates of MRI and CT Services for Select Provider Specialties

| Specialty[a] | Percentage of MRI services self-referred in 2004 | Percentage of MRI services self-referred in 2010 | Change in MRI Self-referral rate from 2004 to 2010 (percentage points) | Percentage of CT services self-referred in 2004 | Percentage of CT services self-referred in 2010 | Change in CT self-referral rate from 2004 to 2010 (percentage points) |
|---|---|---|---|---|---|---|
| Cardiology | n/a | n/a | n/a | 33.5 % | 55.4% | 21.9 |
| Family Practice | 10.8 | 15.7 | 4.8 | 25.0 | 27.6 | 2.6 |
| Gastroenterology | n/a | n/a | n/a | 18.5 | 24.0 | 5.5 |
| General Surgery | n/a | n/a | n/a | 21.5 | 24.8 | 3.3 |
| Hematology/Oncology | 15.3 | 34.3 | 19.0 | 39.8 | 48.7 | 9.0 |
| Internal Medicine | 12.1 | 16.1 | 4.0 | 27.2 | 29.0 | 1.8 |
| Medical Oncology | n/a | n/a | n/a | 39.7 | 51.7 | 12.0 |
| Neurology | 19.7 | 28.9 | 9.1 | n/a | n/a | n/a |
| Neurosurgery | 20.5 | 26.1 | 5.6 | n/a | n/a | n/a |
| Physical Medicine | 22.7 | 29.4 | 6.7 | n/a | n/a | n/a |
| Orthopedic Surgery | 27.1 | 38.4 | 11.4 | n/a | n/a | n/a |
| Otolaryngology | n/a | n/a | n/a | 21.3 | 32.4 | 11.1 |
| Pulmonary Disease | n/a | n/a | n/a | 27.8 | 29.7 | 1.9 |
| Radiation Oncology | n/a | n/a | n/a | 37.7 | 76.1 | 38.4 |
| Rheumatology | 29.4 | 38.6 | 9.2 | n/a | n/a | n/a |
| Urology | n/a | n/a | n/a | 27.8 | 51.2 | 23.4 |

Source: GAO analysis of Medicare data.

Notes: "n/a" indicates that the provider specialty referred less than1.5 percent of all self-referred services, for MRI or CT services, in either 2004 or 2010. If a provider specialty did not refer at least 1.5 percent of all self-referred services for both 2004 and 2010 for either MRI or CT services, it is not included in the table.

[a]Provider specialties are included in Medicare claims data and are self-reported.

# Appendix IV: Comments from the Department of Health and Human Services

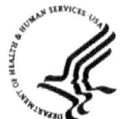

DEPARTMENT OF HEALTH & HUMAN SERVICES    OFFICE OF THE SECRETARY

Assistant Secretary for Legislation
Washington, DC 20201

**SEP 1 7 2012**

James Cosgrove
Director, Health Care
U.S. Government Accountability Office
441 G Street NW
Washington, DC  20548

Dear Mr. Cosgrove:

Attached are comments on the U.S. Government Accountability Office's (GAO) report entitled,
"MEDICARE: Higher Use of Advanced Imaging Services by Providers Who Self-Refer Costing
Medicare Millions" (GAO-12-966).

The Department appreciates the opportunity to review this report prior to publication.

Sincerely,

Jim R. Esquea
Assistant Secretary for Legislation

Attachment

GENERAL COMMENTS OF THE DEPARTMENT OF HEALTH AND HUMAN
SERVICES (HHS) ON THE GOVERNMENT ACCOUNTABILITY OFFICE'S (GAO)
DRAFT REPORT ENTITLED, "MEDICARE: HIGHER USE OF ADVANCED
IMAGING SERVICES BY PROVIDERS WHO SELF-REFER COSTING MEDICARE
MILLIONS" (GAO-12-966)

The Department appreciates the opportunity to review and respond to the GAO draft report
entitled, "Higher Use of Advanced Imaging Services by Providers Who Self-Refer Costing
Medicare Millions" (GAO-12-966). We appreciate GAO's efforts to analyze overall trends in
billing by physicians who self-refer and the impact that it has on Medicare expenditures under
Part B.

The Social Security Act (the Act) currently includes provisions that address when physicians
may own certain diagnostic and therapeutic equipment and self-refer to furnish those services.
The Stark Law prohibits physicians from making referrals for certain designated health services
paid for by Medicare, to entities with which the physicians or immediate family members have a
financial relationship, unless the arrangement complies with a specified exception, such as for in-
office ancillary services.

Section 1848(c) of the Act requires the Secretary to determine relative values for physicians'
services under the Physician Fee Schedule (PFS) based on physician, work practice expense, and
malpractice. Specifically, the Secretary must consider the relative resources used in providing
the service. Our long standing valuation methodology for the PFS is to assess the resources
involved with furnishing the service for the "typical" case. The Medicare statute does not permit
different payment based on the specialty of the physician that provides the service.

As GAO discusses in this report, CMS already has fully implemented a multiple procedure
payment reduction (MPPR) on the technical component of certain diagnostic advanced imaging
procedures. CMS adopted a 25 percent transitional reduction that the Affordable Care Act later
increased to 50 percent effective July 2010. The reduction for the second and subsequent
imaging procedure took into consideration clinical labor, supplies, and equipment time that
would be duplicated if full payment were made for all services in the typical case. In response to
GAO and Medicare Payment Advisory Commission recommendations, CMS extended the
MPPR on diagnostic imaging in 2012 to the physician interpretation or the professional
component of the diagnostic test. The reduction is 25 percent for second and subsequent
procedures furnished by the same physician to the same patient in the same session on the same
day, and we determined that reduction by a review of the physician work involved in the typical
case.

The GAO recommendations and HHS's response to those recommendations are discussed below.

**GAO Recommendation 1**

In order to improve CMS's ability to identify self-referred advanced imaging services and help
CMS address the increases in these services, GAO recommends that the Administrator of CMS
insert a self-referral flag on its Medicare Part B claims form and require providers to indicate
whether the advanced imaging services for which a provider bills Medicare are self-referred or
not.

1

**GENERAL COMMENTS OF THE DEPARTMENT OF HEALTH AND HUMAN
SERVICES (HHS) ON THE GOVERNMENT ACCOUNTABILITY OFFICE'S (GAO)
DRAFT REPORT ENTITLED, "MEDICARE: HIGHER USE OF ADVANCED
IMAGING SERVICES BY PROVIDERS WHO SELF-REFER COSTING MEDICARE
MILLIONS" (GAO-12-966)**

**HHS Response**

HHS does not concur. CMS does not believe this or the GAO's other recommendations will
address overutilization that occurs as a result of self-referral. CMS believes that a new checkbox
on the claim form identifying self-referral would be complex to administer and could have some
unintended consequences (e.g., when a prohibited referral occurs outside the group or clinic
context, the claim will say it's not "self-referred," but it would nevertheless be a referral that
violated the Stark Law). CMS believes other payment reforms such as Accountable Care
Organizations and value-based purchasing programs such as the physician value-based modifier
will better address overutilization than a new checkbox on the claim form that will be complex to
administer and may have unintended consequences for law enforcement.

**GAO Recommendation 2**

GAO recommends that the Administrator of CMS determine and implement a payment reduction
for self-referred advanced imaging services to recognize efficiencies when the same provider
refers and performs a service.

**HHS Response**

HHS does not concur. We note that CMS's multiple procedure payment reduction policy for
advanced imaging already captures efficiencies inherent in providing multiple advanced imaging
services by the same physician or group practice in the same session irrespective of whether
those services are self-referred or not. Moreover, CMS does not believe a further payment
reduction would be effective for two reasons. First, a payment reduction would not address the
underlying conflict of interest that is believed to result in overutilization and higher program
costs. At best, a payment reduction would merely reduce, but not eliminate, the financial
incentive to refer for these services; at worst, it would incentivize physicians to maintain their
income from such services by referring for even more imaging services, resulting in little or no
change in program costs and possibly reduced quality of care. Second, such a payment reduction
could be easily avoided if one physician in a practice were to order the service while another
physician in the same practice were to furnish the service. Finally, CMS questions its statutory
authority to impose the payment reduction suggested by GAO. The Medicare statute prohibits
paying a differential by physician specialty for the same service. While the multiple payment
procedure reduction reduces payment for all physicians when they perform multiple services in a
single session, GAO's recommendation would make different payment for a single service based
on whether a physician has a financial interest in the service being referred and ordered.

2

**GENERAL COMMENTS OF THE DEPARTMENT OF HEALTH AND HUMAN
SERVICES (HHS) ON THE GOVERNMENT ACCOUNTABILITY OFFICE'S (GAO)
DRAFT REPORT ENTITLED, "MEDICARE: HIGHER USE OF ADVANCED
IMAGING SERVICES BY PROVIDERS WHO SELF-REFER COSTING MEDICARE
MILLIONS" (GAO-12-966)**

**GAO Recommendation 3**

GAO recommends that the Administrator of CMS determine and implement an approach to
ensure the appropriateness of advanced imaging services referred by self-referring providers.

**HHS Response**

CMS will consider this recommendation when refining its medical review strategy for advanced
imaging services. We note that CMS does not have the statutory authority to implement some of
the approaches discussed in the report, such as prior authorization for self-referred imaging
services.

3

# Appendix V: GAO Contact and Staff Acknowledgments

| | |
|---|---|
| **GAO Contact** | James C. Cosgrove, (202) 512-7114 or cosgrovej@gao.gov |
| **Staff Acknowledgments** | In addition to the contact named above, Jessica Farb, Assistant Director; Thomas Walke, Assistant Director; Manuel Buentello; Krister Friday; Gregory Giusto; Brian O'Donnell; and Daniel Ries made key contributions to this report. |